The Publishers thank the Staff of the West Middlesex Hospital, and Nancy Safford, Honorary Secretary of the National Association for the Welfare of Children in Hospital for their assistance in the preparation of this book.

 Based on an idea by Judith Burnley and illustrated by Julie Simpson. First published in Great Britain in 1973 by Studio Vista Publishers, Blue Star House, Highgate Hill, London N 19. Filmset by BAS Printers Limited, Wallop. Printed by Colour Reproductions Limited, Billericay, and bound by R. J. Acford Limited, Chichester.
ISBN (paperback) 0 289 70367 0 (hard bound) 0 289 70368 9

come inside the HOSPITAL

Julie Simpson

Studio Vista London

The hospital was a group of large, grey buildings. One Saturday afternoon, Peter and his father went there to see Peter's mother who had just had a baby.

Outside the main entrance they stopped to look at a sign-post. Peter's father read out some of the names: 'Out-patients, Accident and Emergency, X-Ray, Operating Theatre, Medical Ward, Surgical Ward, Plaster Room, Pharmacy, Physiotherapy Department, Maternity Ward.'

'Where's Mummy?' asked Peter.

'She's in the Maternity Ward,' replied his father. 'That's the name of the place where mothers have their babies. Shall we buy Mummy some flowers?'

Peter and his father each bought a big bunch of flowers from a man who had a flower-stall just outside the swing doors of the hospital entrance.

'You give yours to Mummy and I'll give mine to the baby,' said Peter.

Peter's father asked a nurse, who was hurrying along, if they were going the right way.

'Yes,' she said, looking at the watch pinned to her white apron. 'But take your time because she will just be waking up now and having a cup of tea. All the mothers sleep in the afternoons as they have to feed their babies late at night and very early in the morning.'

Peter and his father thanked her and went through the big entrance doors. Inside was a large hall with lots of people hurrying about. There were visitors carrying bunches of flowers and bags of fruit, doctors in white coats, nurses in uniform, and two men sitting in a little office.

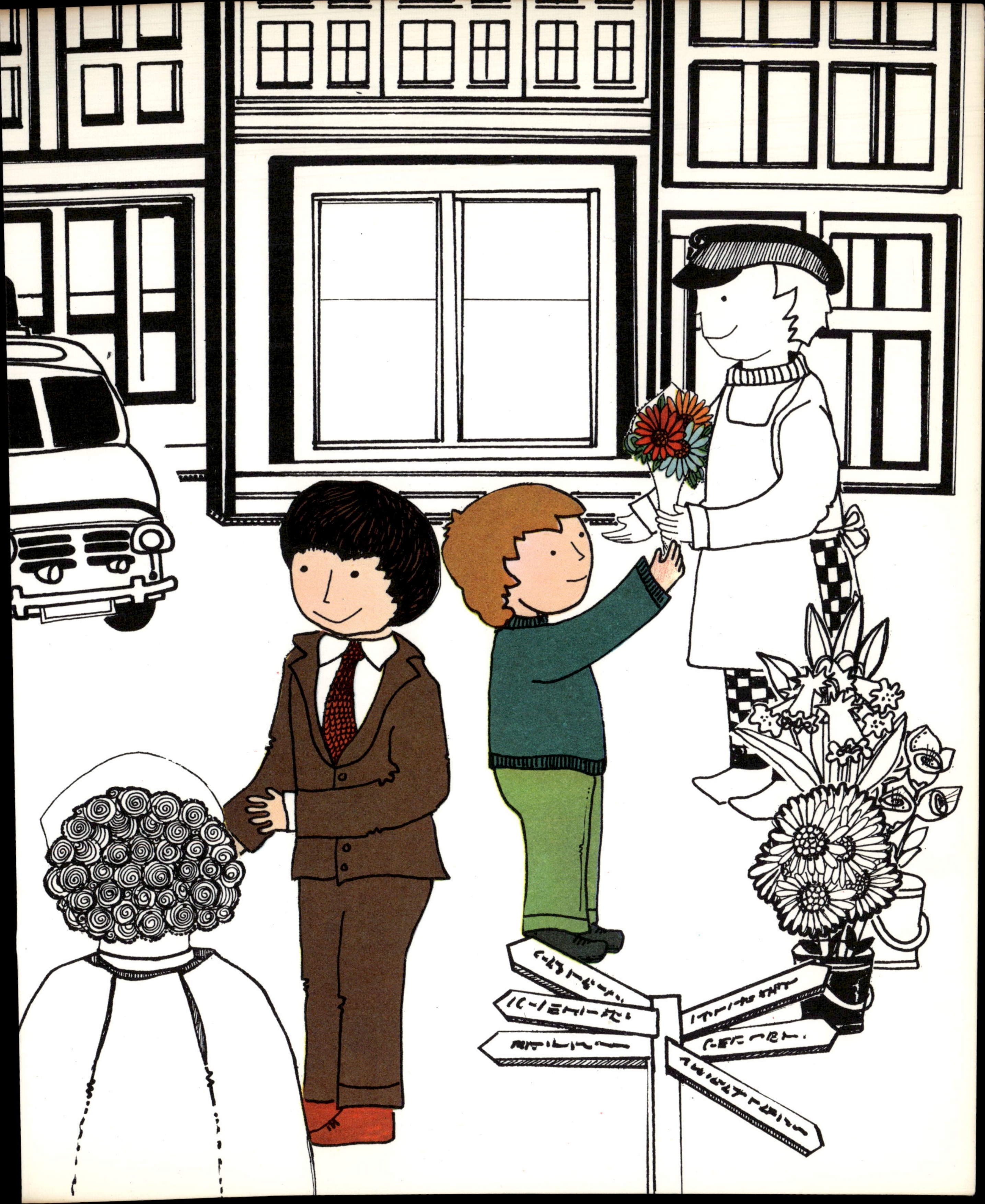

Peter and his father followed the signs to the Maternity Ward. Peter's father was allowed to go in but Peter was asked by a nurse to wait outside for a while. He sat on a chair in the corridor and watched visitors and nurses go in and out of the ward's swing doors. But soon he was bored and decided to explore. The corridor was very wide with doors all along it and busy nurses hurrying in and out. He walked along, looking through the doors when they were opened. He could see people in beds and smiled at them. But they all seemed to be reading or talking to visitors and did not notice him.

Peter walked on to the end of the corridor and turned the corner into another long corridor. It looked the same as the one he had just come from. More doors, more nurses, more people in beds. So he went on to the next corner and the next corridor, and it was the same. He stopped and looked back. Which way had he come? He turned round and looked up the corridor and looked down the corridor, but did not know which way to go.

'What's the matter?' said a voice. 'You look lost.'

Peter looked round. Behind him stood a man in a white coat with a stethoscope round his neck, smiling at him.

'I've lost my mother, father and sister somewhere in all these corridors,' answered Peter.

'What part of the hospital are they in?' asked the man.

'I can't remember the name of it,' said Peter.

'Was it Accident and Emergency?' asked the man.

'I've heard the names before, so it could be,' said Peter.

'Well, come with me and we'll look,' said the man. 'I was on my way there when I saw you.'

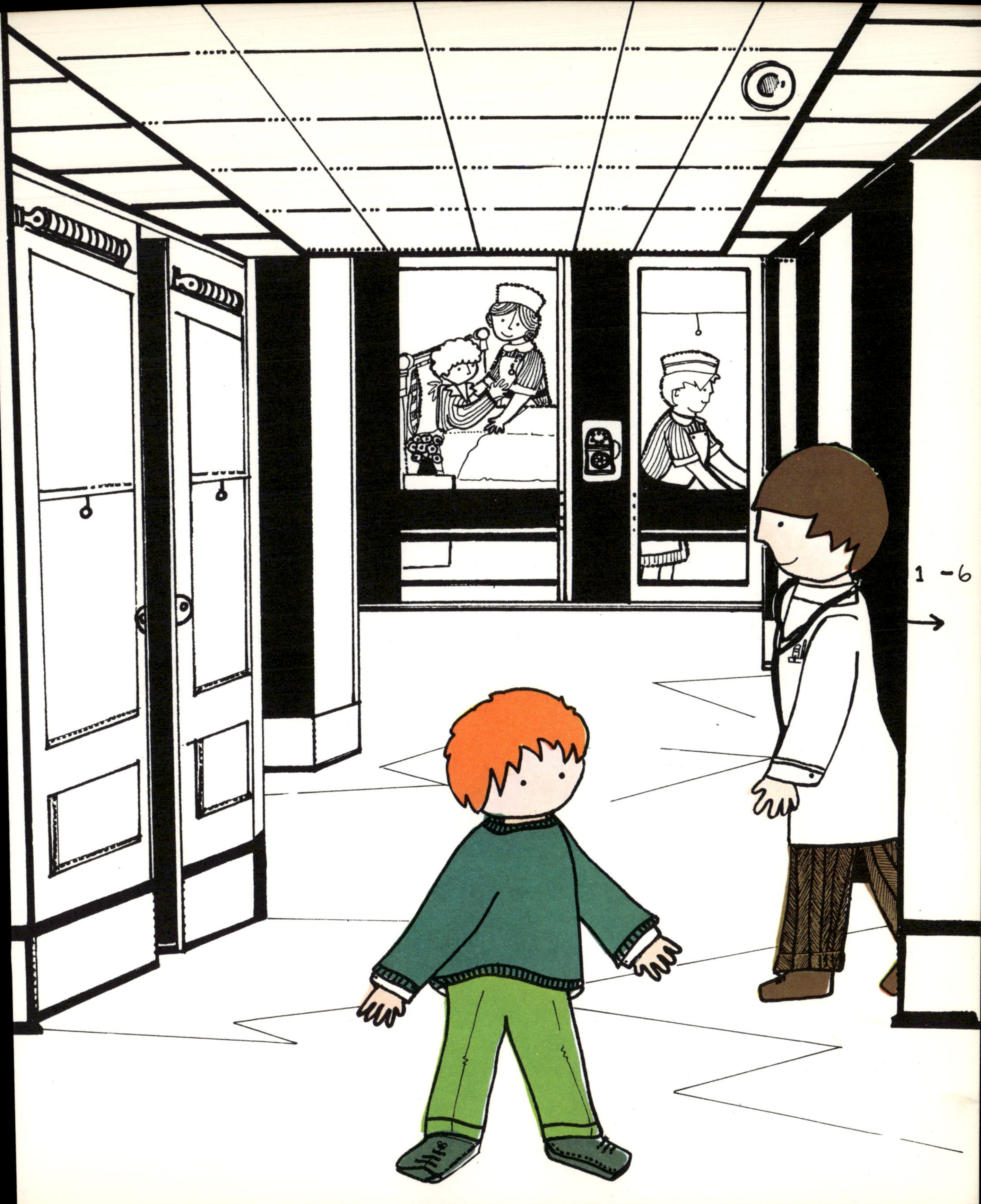
1 -6

Together they walked down the corridors, passing hurrying nurses and porters in white coats pushing trolleys. Everything was very clean and shining.

The man said to Peter: 'I'm a doctor and I work in the hospital. I'm called a houseman. Sometimes I'm here during the night but this week I'm working during the day.'

On the way to the Accident and Emergency Department, they passed a door labelled 'Out-patients'.

'What are Out-patients?' asked Peter.

'They are just what the word says,' replied the houseman. 'They are people who are not ill enough to have to stay in hospital but they need our care and attention. If you look in you can see two boys with their arms in slings. They have come to the Out-patients Department so that the doctor can see if their arms are healing properly.'

Peter looked round the door.

'That boy fell out of a tree and bumped his head,' said the houseman. 'The girl cut her leg and had to have it stitched up. The other boy, with his knee and finger bandaged, fell down in the road when he was running too fast. He has come so that the doctor can change the bandages.'

There were other children sitting on chairs with their mothers, waiting their turn to see the doctor. Some were playing with toys while others were reading.

'We also look after people who have been in hospital and are well enough to go home but just need a little treatment or more medicine,' said the houseman. 'But let's go on to Accident and Emergency.'

'I don't think that can be the right place,' said Peter.

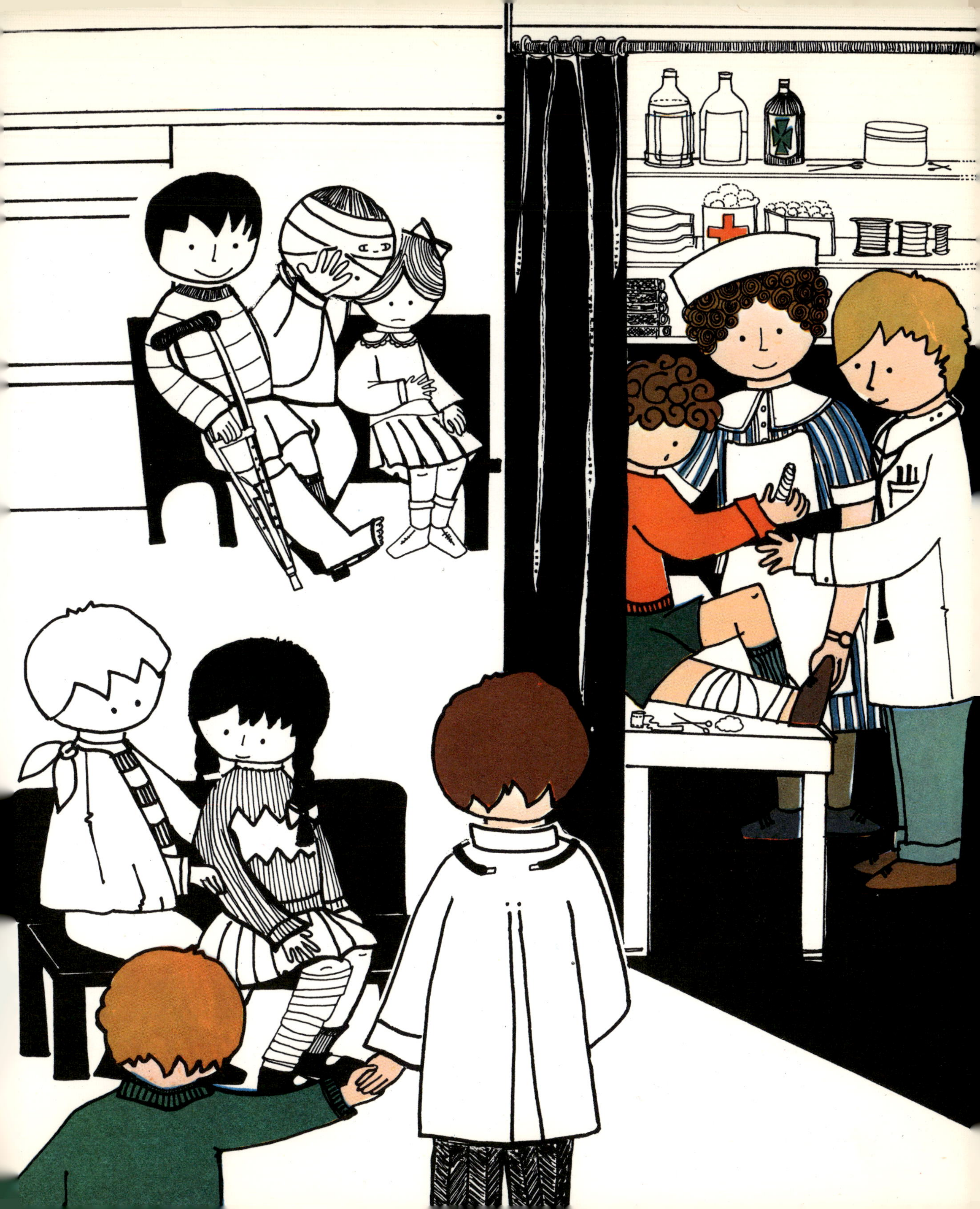

They went on down the corridors, passing doors and turning many corners.

'Accident and Emergency, as the names say, is the place where people who have had accidents or are suddenly taken very ill come for treatment,' said the houseman. 'If they are not badly hurt, they can go home after they have been treated by the doctor and nurses. If they have had a very bad accident or are very ill, they have to stay in hospital until they are better.'

When they reached Accident and Emergency, Peter and the houseman heard a siren wailing outside. The doors opened and Peter could see an ambulance. Two ambulance-men in uniform carefully lifted a stretcher out of the ambulance and carried it into the Department. On it lay a boy, wrapped in a warm blanket.

'He ran across a road without looking first and was knocked down by a car,' said one of the ambulancemen.

They lifted the boy gently from the stretcher on to a long trolley. A nurse held his hand.

'It's all right,' she said. 'We'll look after you and your mother will be here soon.'

Peter watched as the trollcy was wheeled away.

'Where are they taking him?' he asked.

'Into an examination room,' replied the houseman, 'so that the doctor can look at him and find out if he has been badly hurt. And decide what treatment he needs to make him better. You can watch if you like.'

With the houseman, Peter walked along a corridor and into the examination room.

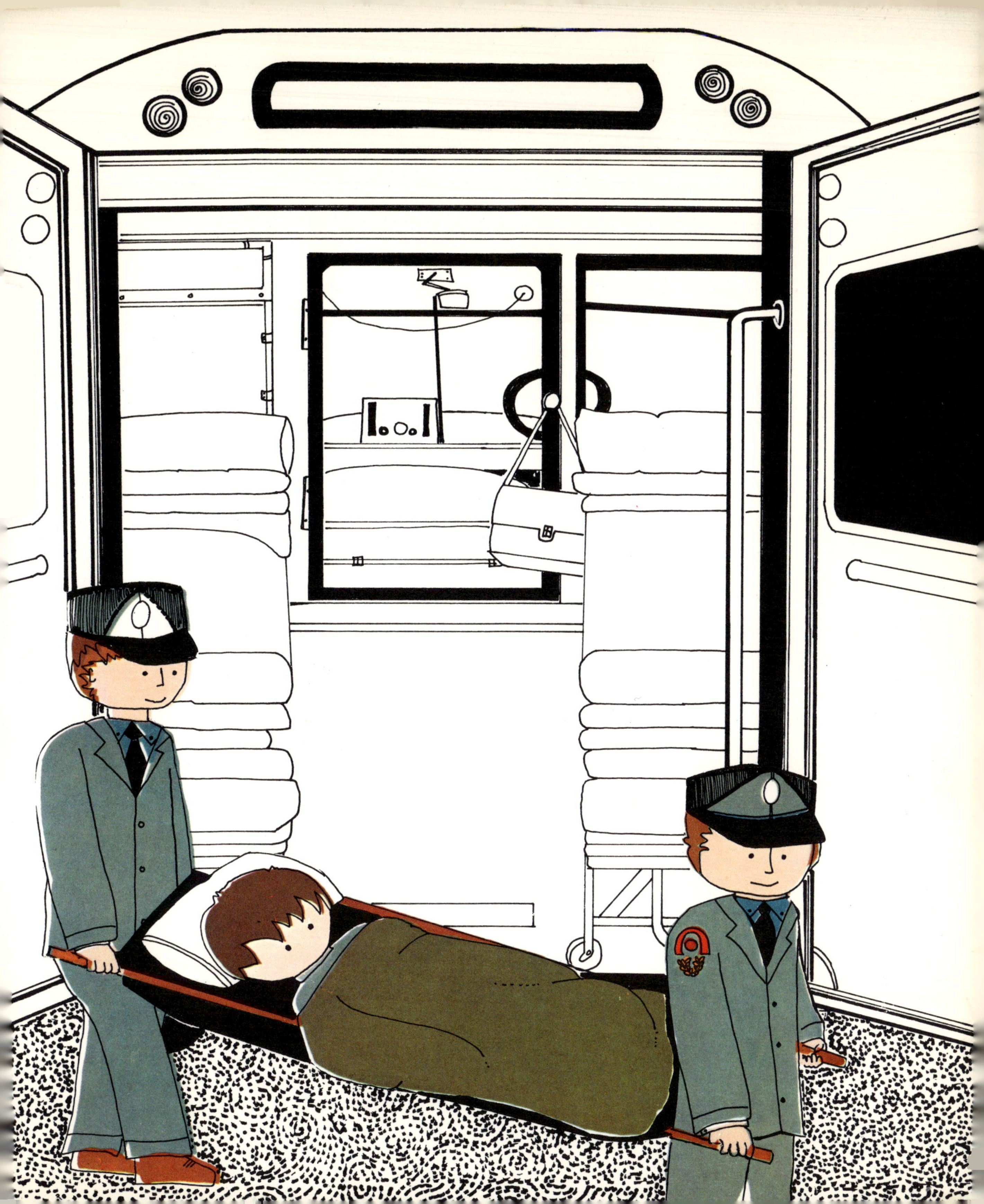

The examination room was very brightly lit. Round the walls were shelves full of instruments and bottles and baskets of rolled bandages.

The doctor in a white coat looked carefully at the boy. Then he rolled up one of the boy's sleeves.

'I'm going to give you an injection,' he said. 'It will stop things hurting for a while. You will feel the little prick of the needle but it will soon be over so try to be a brave boy.'

The doctor dipped a piece of cotton wool into some antiseptic and rubbed a small place on the boy's arm.

'After I've given you the injection,' the doctor said, 'we're going to take you for another ride on the trolley to the X-ray department. And we'll find out if any of your bones have been broken.'

The boy looked a little happier.

'Can I go home then?' he asked.

'Well, we'll see,' said the nurse. 'You may have to stay in hospital for a few days. But you would be in a children's ward and your mother would visit you every day.'

Peter watched the doctor give the boy the injection. Then a porter in a white coat pushed the trolley out through the doors of the examination room and along the corridor.

'My mother hasn't had an accident,' said Peter, 'so she won't be here. But I've heard of X-ray before so perhaps she's there.'

'Let's go and look,' answered the houseman. 'You are not allowed to go into the X-ray department but you can look through the window in the door for her. And you can see what happens to this brave boy here.'

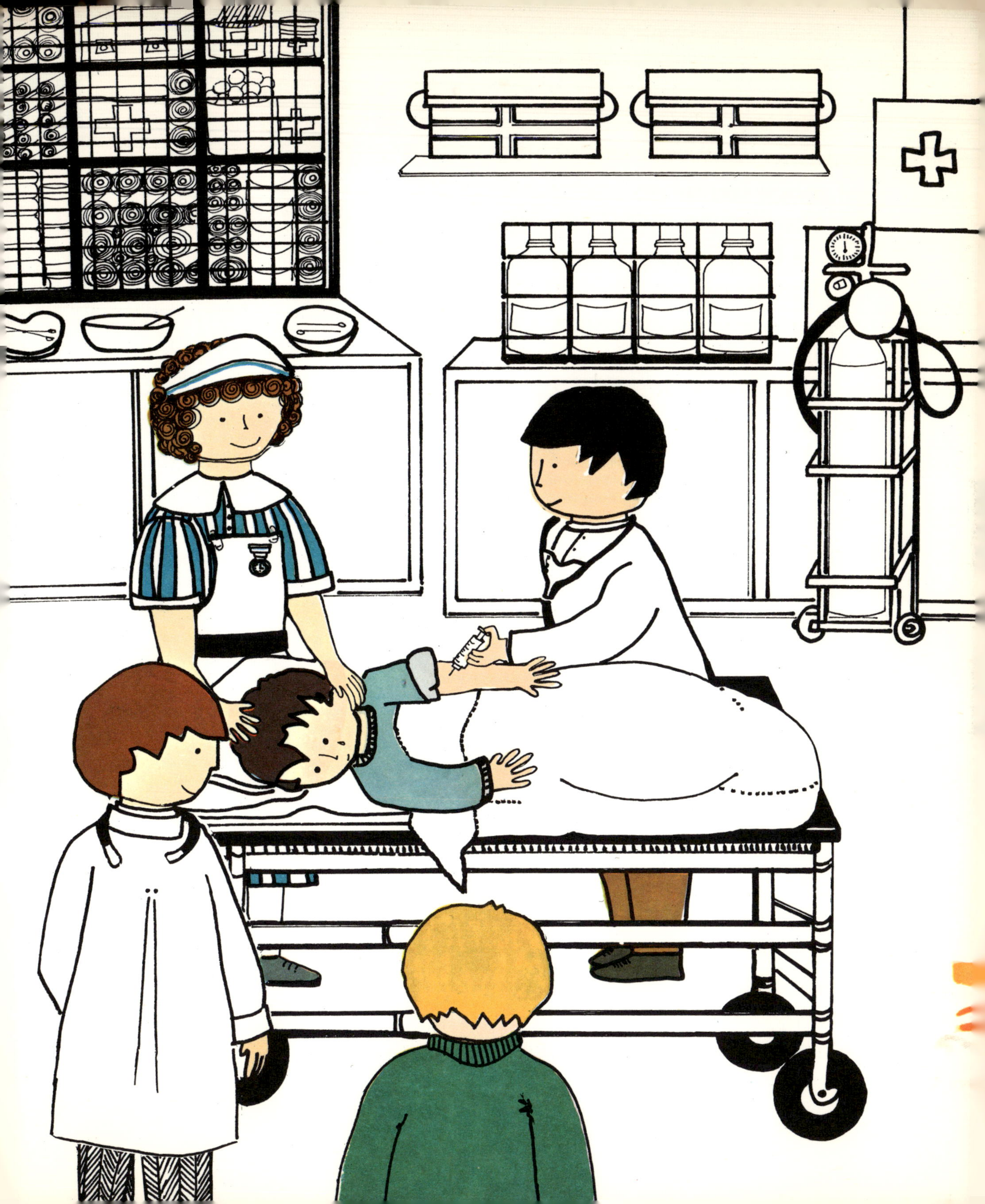

In the X-ray room, Peter saw the boy lying on a long padded table. There were strange machines round him and a huge one suspended over the table.

'What's happening to him?' Peter asked the houseman.

'They are taking pictures of the boy's bones with a special camera that can see through his skin,' answered the houseman. 'With these pictures we can find if any of the boy's bones are broken.'

'What are the other machines?' Peter asked.

'We have two types of X-ray machine. One type to take special photographs and another for what is called screening. The screening one is a type of camera which puts pictures of someone's insides directly on to a type of television screen.'

The boy had been hit very hard. The X-rays showed that he had a broken arm and a broken leg. He was put on a trolley again and wheeled away.

'Where's he going now?' asked Peter.

'He's going to the Accident Theatre,' said the houseman. 'That's a small operating theatre where the doctor will put his broken bones together in the right places again.'

'Can I watch?' Peter said.

'I'm sorry you can't do that,' replied the houseman. 'The doctor and nurses who go into the operating theatre have to wash very carefully and put on special gowns, shoes and masks so that they don't take any germs in. And they have to work very quickly so they couldn't have you in there.'

'Does it hurt when someone's broken bones are put together?' said Peter.

'No,' said the houseman. 'The boy won't feel anything at

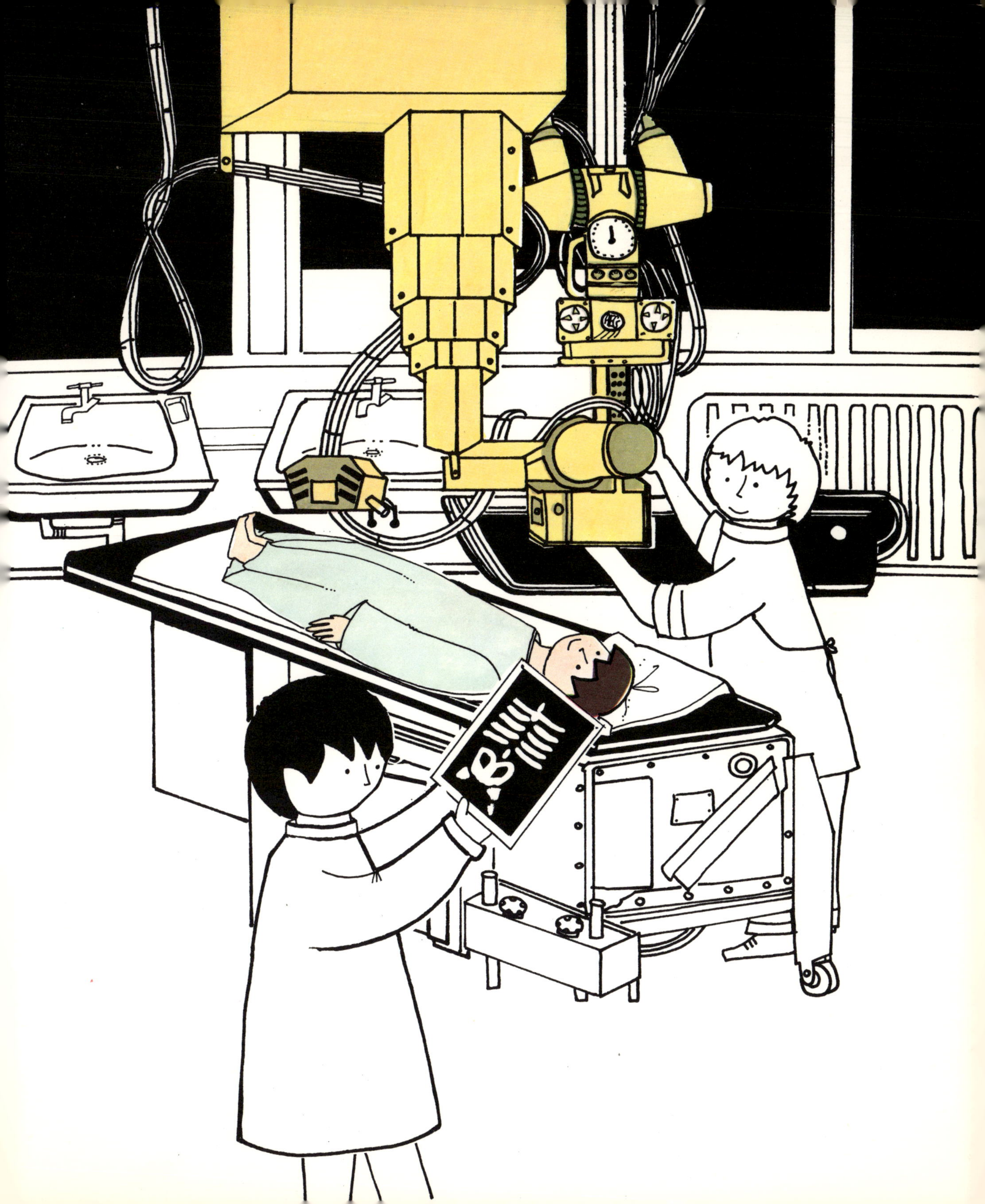

all. The doctor will put the boy to sleep before he is taken into the operating theatre. As well as the doctor and nurses, there's the anaesthetist.'

'What's the anaesthetist?' asked Peter.

'The anaesthetist is the man who puts a mask over the patient's nose so that he breathes in a special gas which makes him sleep all through the operation. The gas is in cylinders on a special trolley and there are dials to show the anaesthetist that the pressure in the cylinders is right. When the patient wakes up, the operation is all over.'

Peter was disappointed that he could not watch the operation so a nurse asked the houseman if she could show Peter an empty operating theatre and then go on with the search for his father and mother.

The nurse dressed Peter in a large overall and put some big plastic shoes on his feet. She changed her shoes too. Then she led him into a white tiled room. Everything was very clean and shining. In the centre of the room was a long table with a huge lamp hanging over it.

'When the surgeons are operating,' said the nurse, 'they need a very good light to shine on the patient lying on the table. Now, where's your mother?'

'She isn't in Out-patients, or Accident and Emergency, or X-ray. And she didn't need an operation,' said Peter.

'Well, she might be in the Medical Ward then,' said the nurse.

'I've heard that name before,' said Peter. 'Are there any children in the Medical Ward. I have a baby sister.'

'She could be there,' said the nurse. 'Let's look.'

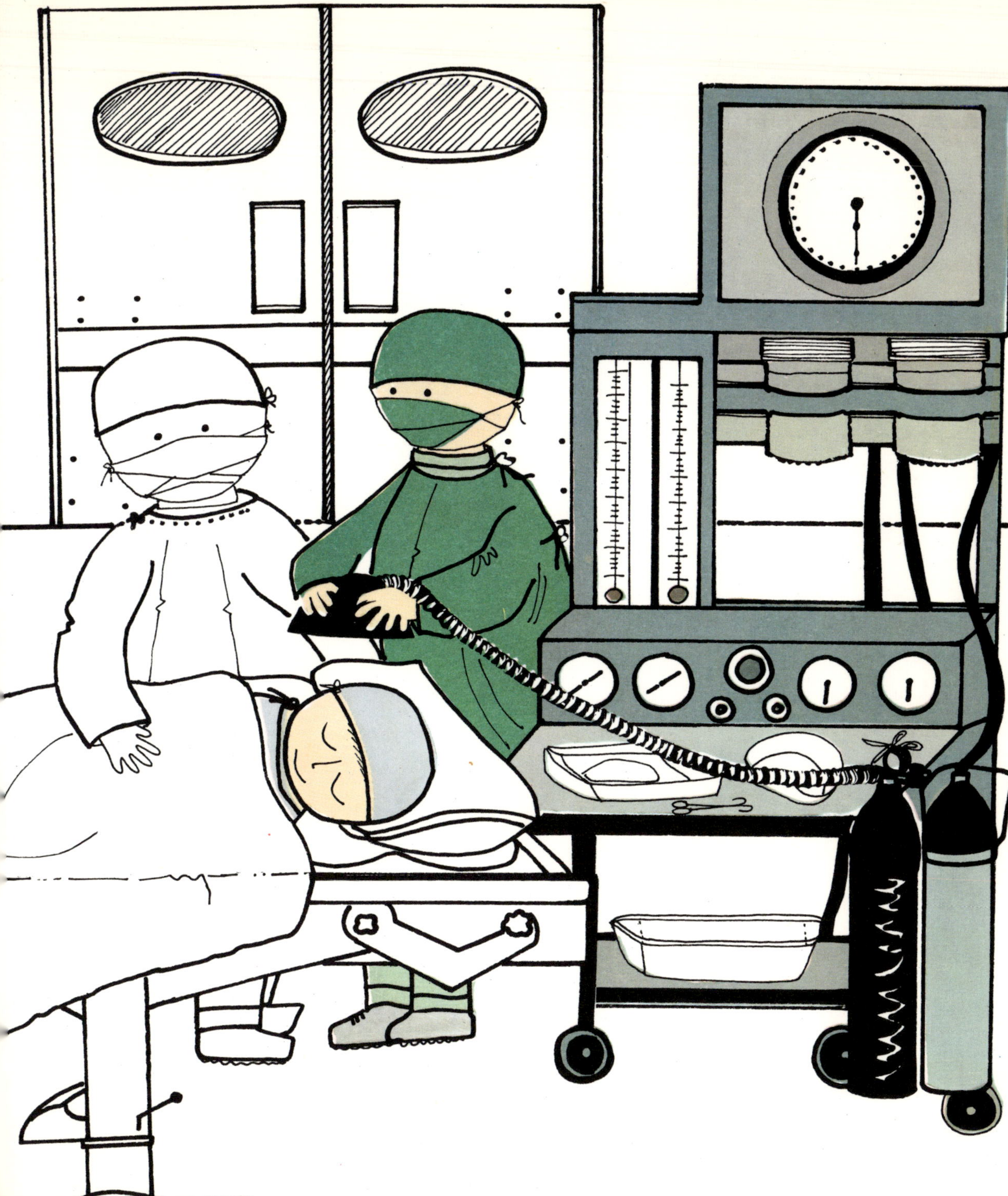

In the Medical ward there were separate rooms, some with one bed and some with three or four beds.

'Some patients have to be on their own if they are very ill or have an infection which other patients can catch,' said the nurse. 'This ward is mainly for people who have some sort of infection.'

Peter looked through the glass walls at a little girl. She lay in bed and a tube, bandaged to her arm, led to a bottle hanging on a stand.

'What's the matter with her?' he asked.

'She's too ill to eat,' said the nurse, 'so we are giving her liquid food through the tube until she is better.'

Peter noticed that her teddybear had a tube bandaged to his arm too.

'She was a bit frightened of the tube until she saw that her teddybear had one as well,' said the nurse.

Peter looked through the windows of the other rooms. Some children were reading or playing or sleeping but they all looked quite happy.

'My sister isn't here,' said Peter. 'She isn't in Medical.'

'Let's try children's Surgical then,' said the nurse.

The Surgical Ward was bright and cheerful. There was a television set, bright pictures on the walls and, at one end, tables and chairs for the children who were well enough to get out of bed. Some children were colouring books or painting, some were doing puzzles and some were reading.

'Why is your leg tied up?' Peter asked a boy whose leg was in plaster and hanging by a web of wires and metal weights.

'I'm in traction,' said the boy. 'I broke my leg very badly.

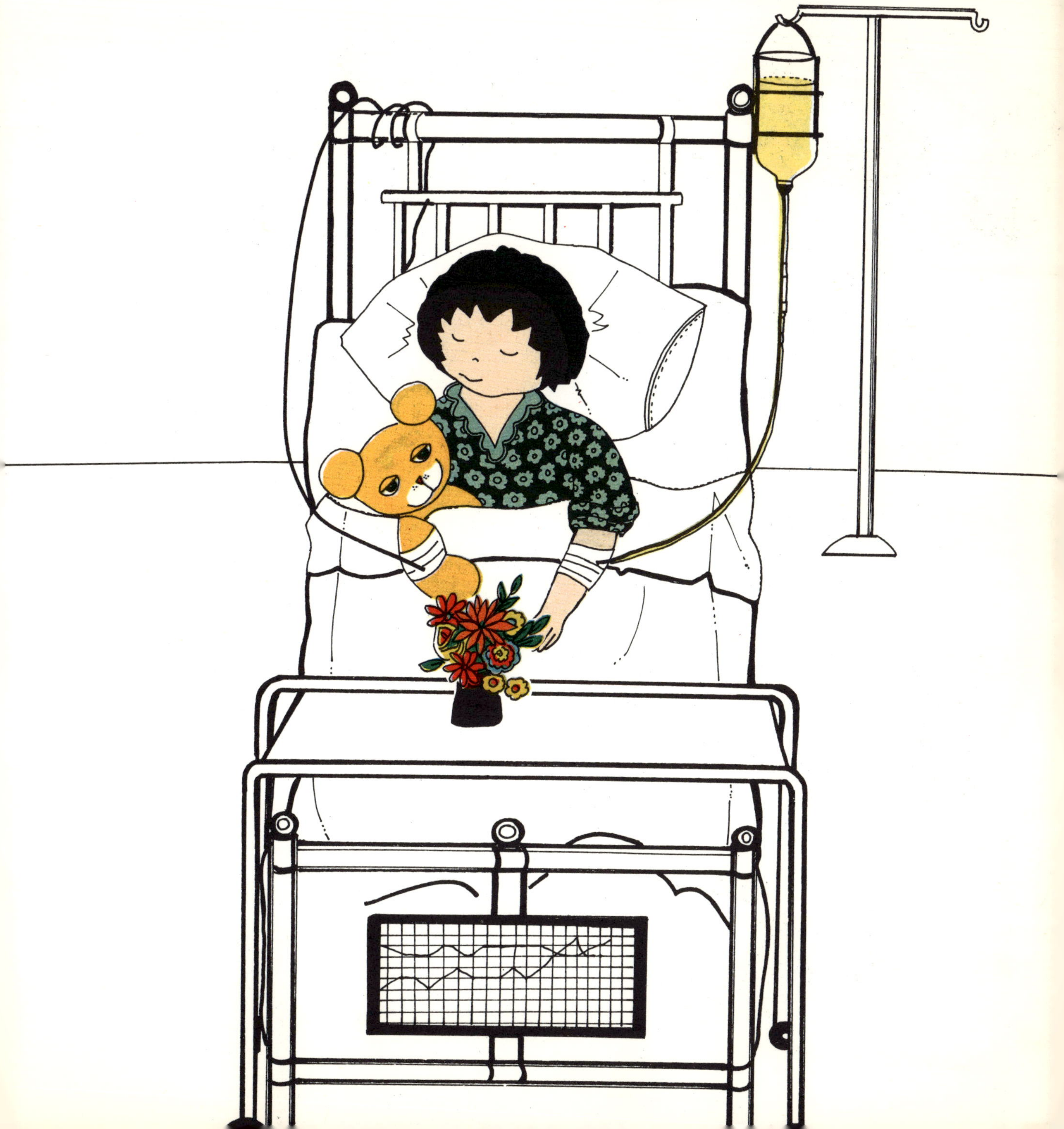

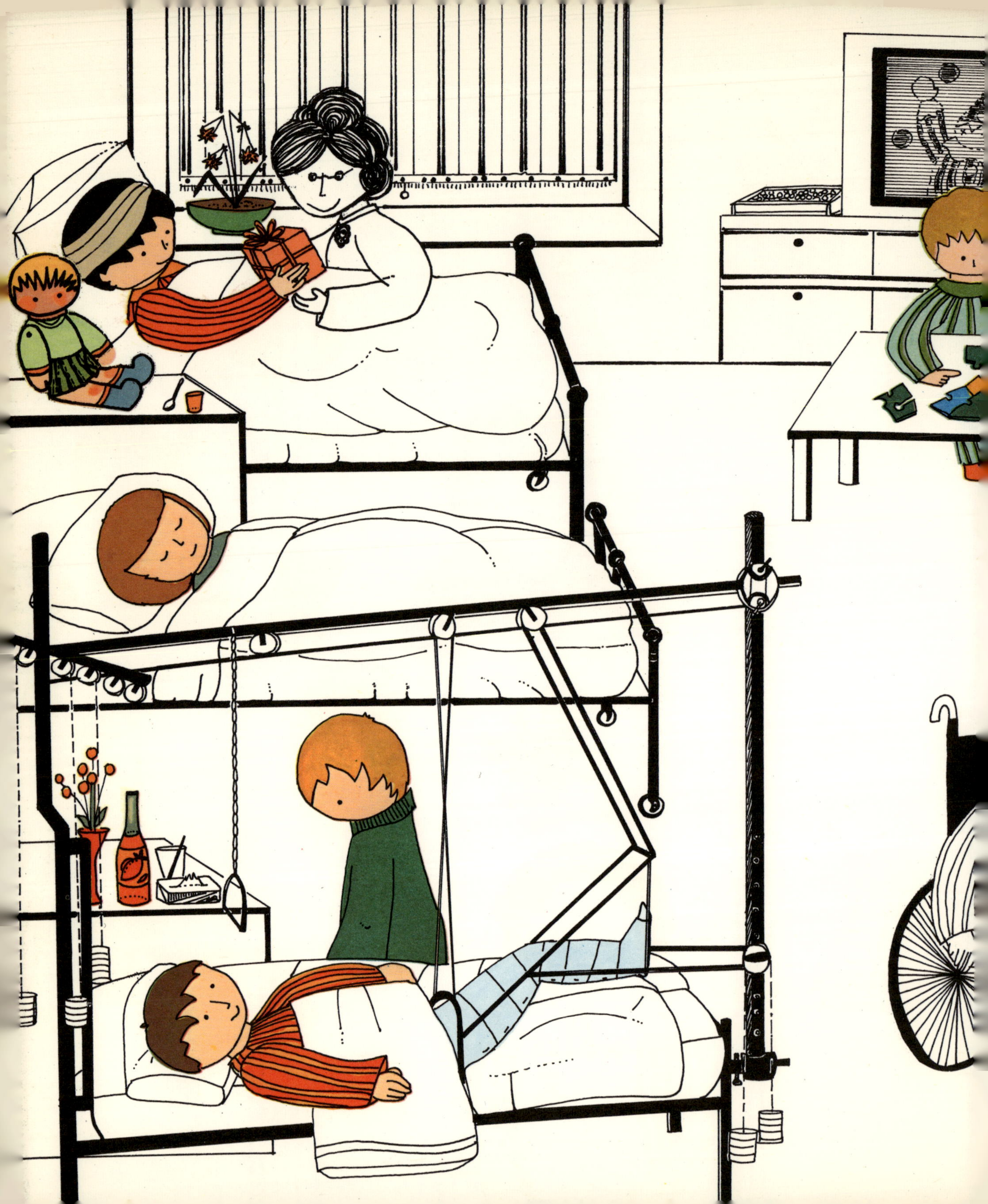

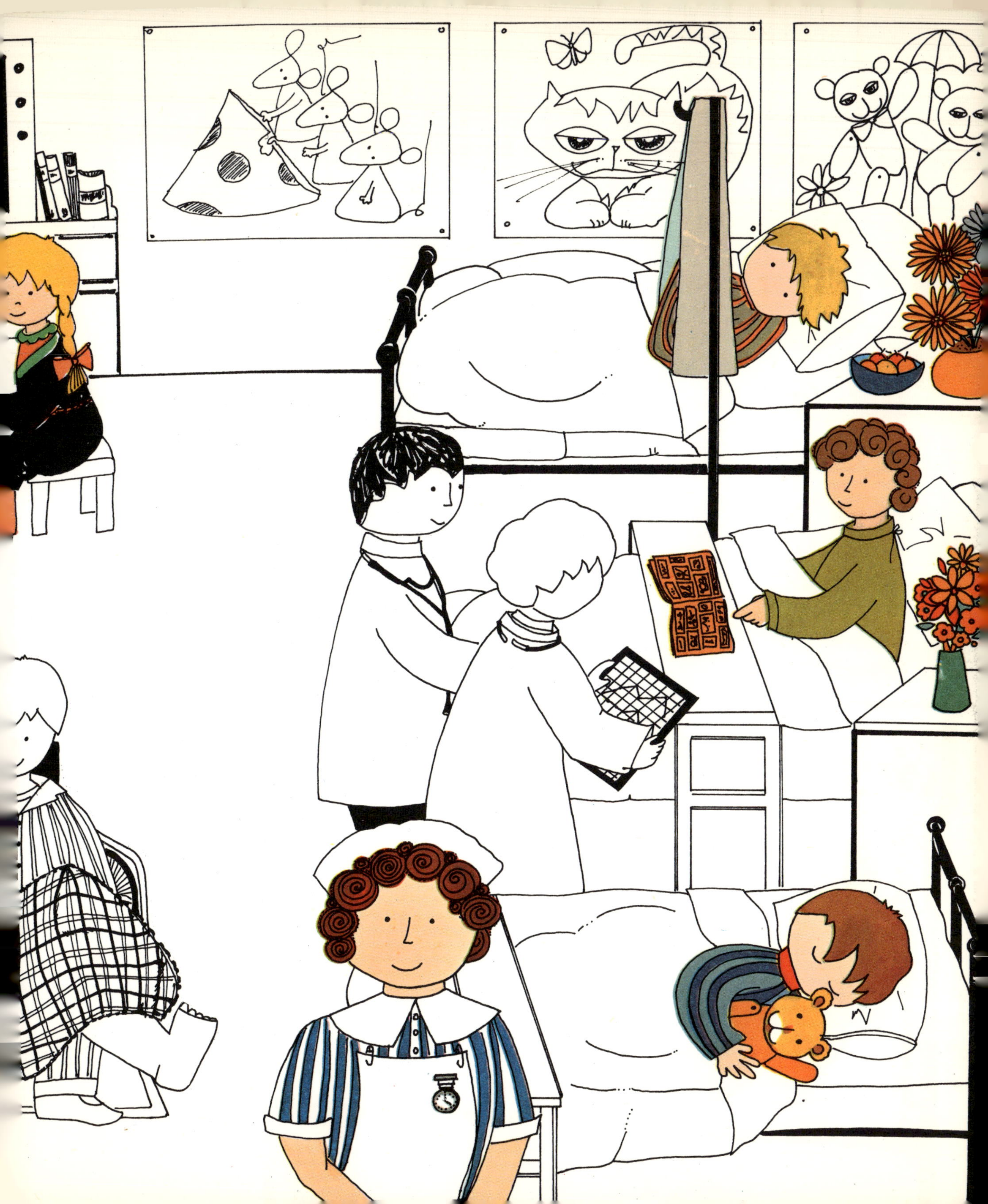

It has to be kept straight and steady while the bones knit together again. It looks funny but it's quite comfortable.'

The nurse put her head round the door. 'Have you found your sister, Peter?' she asked. She was pushing a metal trolley loaded with plates of hot food.

'My sister is not a Surgical case,' said Peter.

'I'm going to the kitchens now to check a special diet,' said the nurse. 'Then I'm going to the Pharmacy. Do you want to come with me?'

In the kitchens there were huge cookers and ovens and machines for preparing vegetables.

'When the meals are ready,' said the nurse, 'the cooks fill the plates with hot food. The plates are then covered and put on to trolleys which are wheeled quickly to the wards.'

She pointed to the end of the kitchens.

'That is a separate section where the special diets are cooked for patients who can't eat ordinary food.'

Then the nurse hurried Peter to the Pharmacy. The room was lined with shelves full of bottles of liquids and powders. One woman was counting pills into bottles. Another was measuring and mixing powders. She put them into a machine and they came out as pills. A man was working a machine which filled tubes with ointment and then sealed the ends.

'When a doctor wants a patient to have some medicine,' said the man, 'he writes a note called a prescription. He sends it here and we mix up the medicine. Then we write the patient's name and how often he is take the medicine on a label, stick it on the bottle and send it to the ward.'

'I'm going now to the Plaster Room and Physiotherapy,

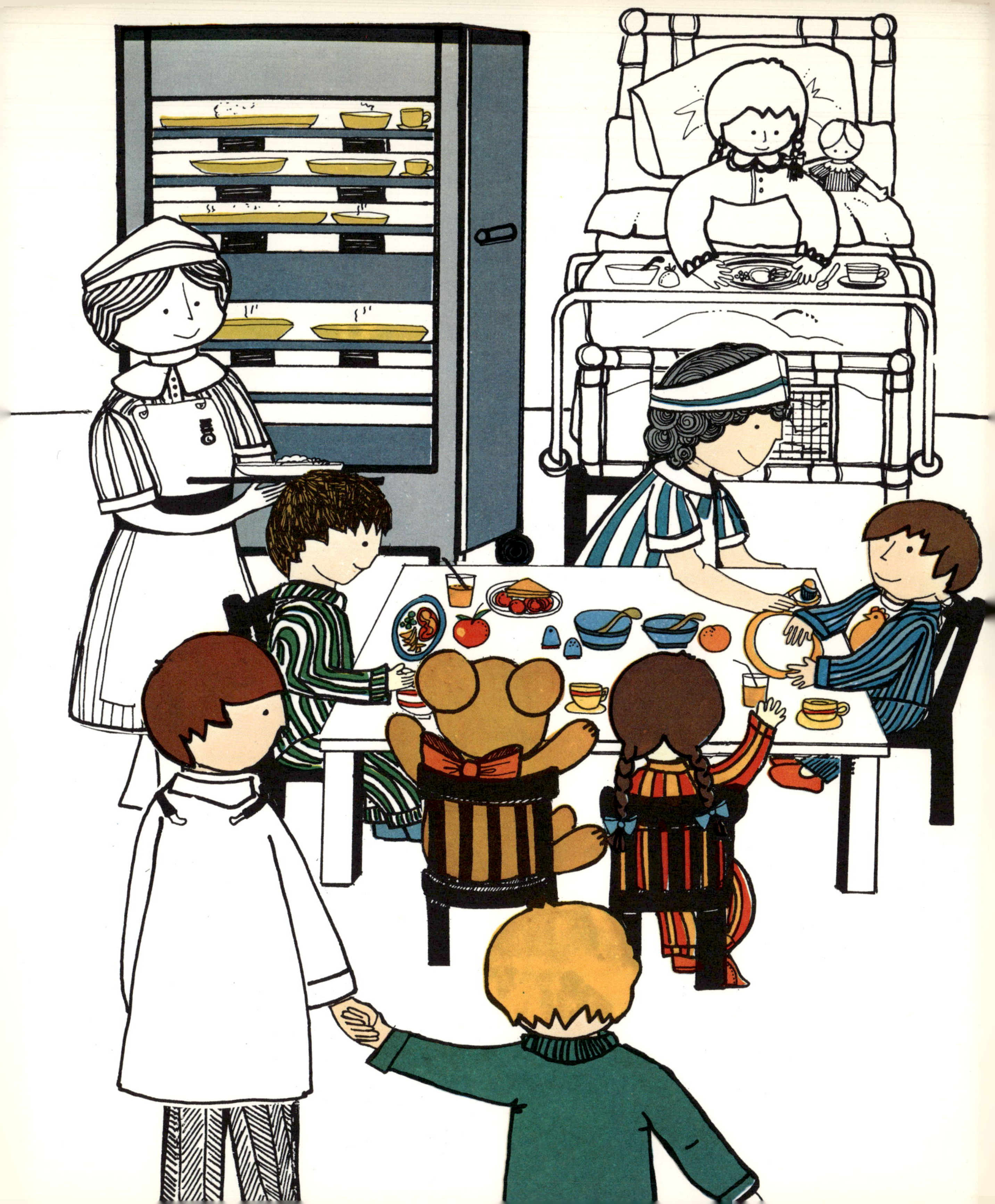

Peter,' said the nurse. 'I don't suppose your mother and sister will be there, but we'll look all the same.'

In the Plaster Room a cheerful man in a white coat was talking to a small boy who had one leg in plaster.

'Which do you want off, the plaster or the leg?' he asked.

'I'd rather have the plaster off,' said the boy, laughing.

The man switched on a little electric saw. The boy looked rather worried.

'It can't hurt you,' said the man. 'It's quite safe.'

With the saw, he cut neatly down the plaster. Then he pulled open the plaster and took it off.

'Oh,' said the boy. 'My leg feels so light and cold now.'

'Everyone feels like that when they have a plaster off,' laughed the man. 'But the bone in your leg isn't quite mended yet so I'll have to put a new plaster on.'

'Bother,' said the boy. 'I can't run properly with it on.'

'It won't be for long now,' said the man.

He wrapped the boy's leg with cotton wool. Then he dipped some plaster bandages in a bowl of water and wound them round and round the boy's leg, smoothing out the plaster and working it to the shape of the leg. When he had put on five or six layers, he fitted a rubber heel to the boy's foot and bound it on with more plaster bandages.

'That will give you something to walk on,' he said.

The plaster dried quickly and was soon quite hard. Then the man helped the boy to stand on his good leg and slipped a crutch under each arm.

'See you soon,' he said to the boy and turned to the nurse. 'And what can we do for this one?'

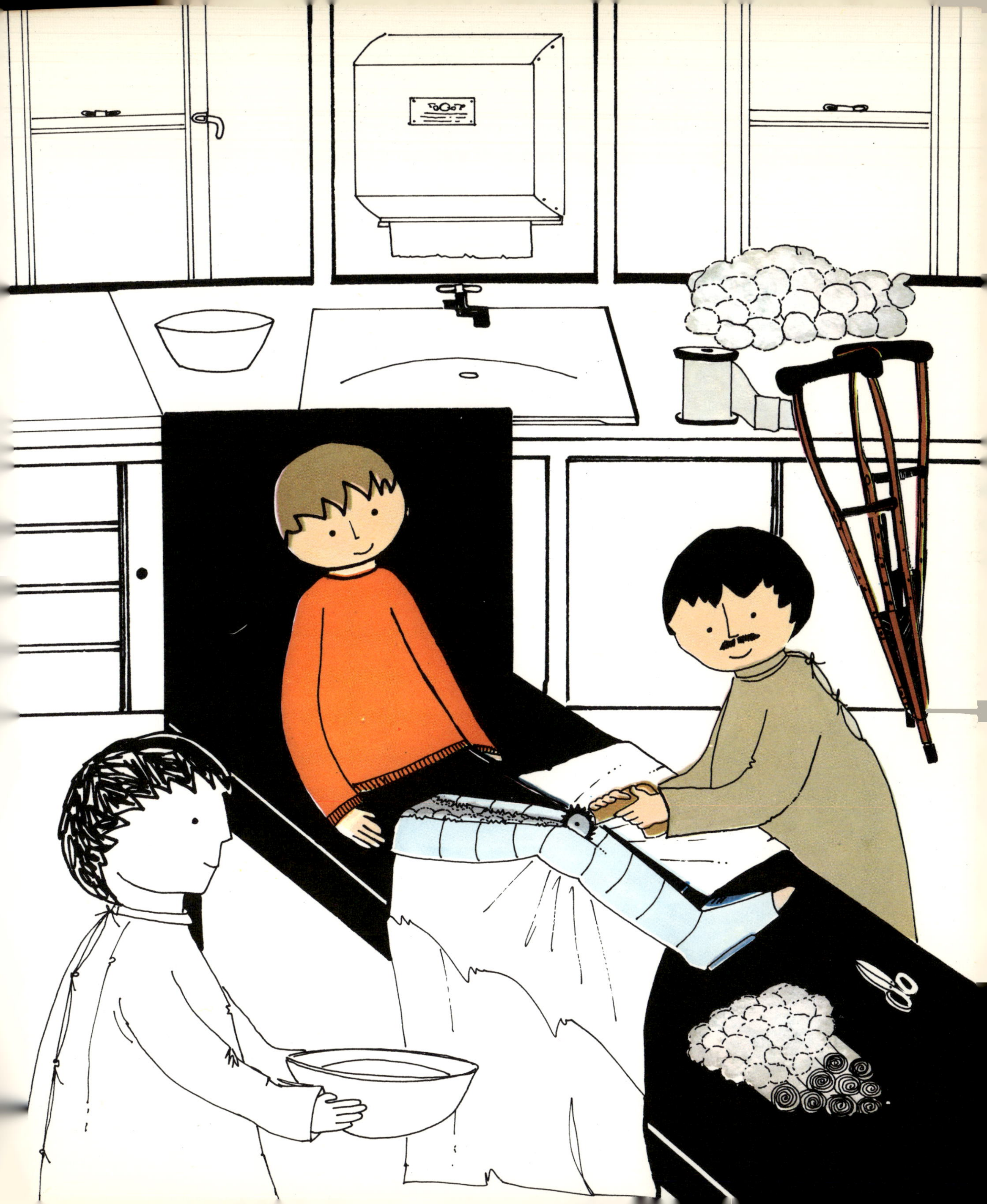

'Nothing with plaster,' answered the nurse, smiling, 'He's lost his father, mother and sister all in one afternoon. We've looked almost all over the hospital and now we're on our way to Physiotherapy.'

Physiotheraphy did not look like part of the hospital at all. It looked like a play room. Children were climbing up wooden wall bars, jumping on a trampoline and balancing along a wooden plank. They were riding rocking horses and tricycles, clapping their hands and playing all sorts of games.

The woman looking after the children explained to Peter: 'These children,' she said, 'are playing with things that exercise weak parts of their bodies and help to make them strong again. Sometimes if a leg has been in plaster for a long time, it gets a bit stiff and needs loosening up. Tricycling is good for stiff knees.'

Everyone looked as if they were enjoying themselves and Peter felt like joining in the fun.

'Some children are doing breathing exercises for chest troubles,' added the woman. 'The little boy pulling on a hoop has a weak left hand which he is trying to make as strong as his right hand.'

'Can you see your sister here?' the nurse asked Peter.

'No,' said Peter. 'She's too young for these games.'

'Why, how old is she?' asked the woman.

'She was born this morning,' answered Peter.

'Born this morning,' said the woman. 'Born this morning,' said the nurse. 'Then we know where your mother is. She's in the Maternity Ward. Let's go there as fast as we can.'

Peter and the nurse almost ran down the corridors and

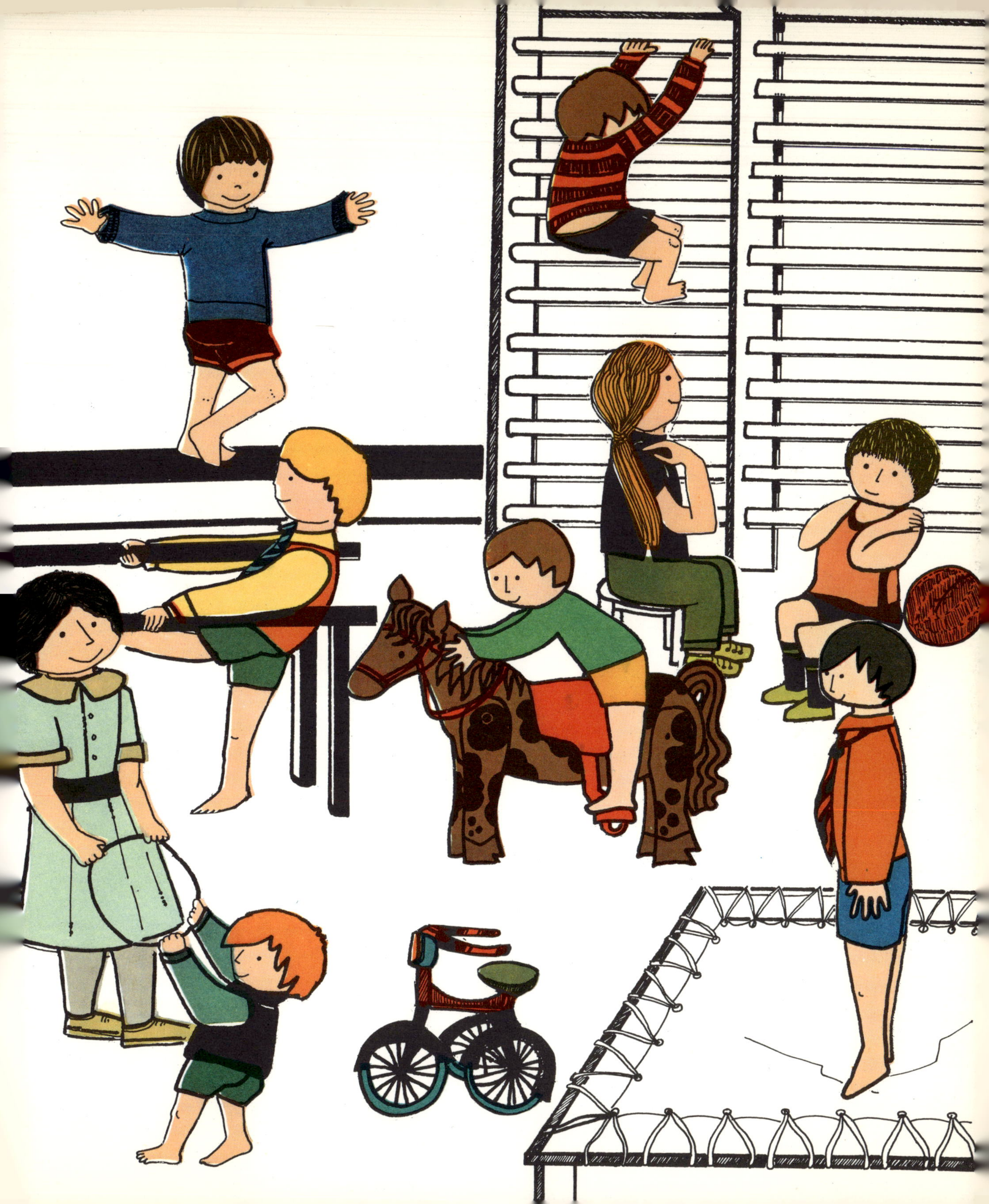

round the corners. When they reached the corridor of the Maternity Ward, they nearly bumped into Peter's father who was looking very worried.

'Is this who you're looking for?' asked the nurse.

Peter's father gave Peter a hug.

'Where have you been?' he asked.

'It's a long story,' said the nurse, smiling.

Peter and his father went into the Maternity Ward. Sitting up in bed, looking very pleased, was Peter's mother. She was holding a small bundle in her arms.

'Oh, Peter,' she cried, 'Daddy has been looking everywhere for you. We were so worried about you. This is your baby sister.' And she held the baby up for him to see.

Peter looked at the baby and smiled. She seemed to be watching him with her bright, unblinking eyes.

'Where have you been?' asked Peter's mother.

'I got lost and looked everywhere for you,' said Peter. 'I've been to Out-patients where people are looked after but can go home. And to Accident and Emergency where injured people come. And to X-ray where they take pictures of your bones and insides. And I've seen an operating theatre. And I've been to the Medical and Surgical Wards, and to the kitchens. And to the Pharmacy where the medicines and pills are made. And to the Plaster Room and to, to, one I can't remember.'

'Physiotherapy,' said the nurse.

'Physiotherapy,' said Peter, 'where you just play all the time and it makes weak parts of your body strong. But, Mummy, I think Maternity is the best ward of all.'

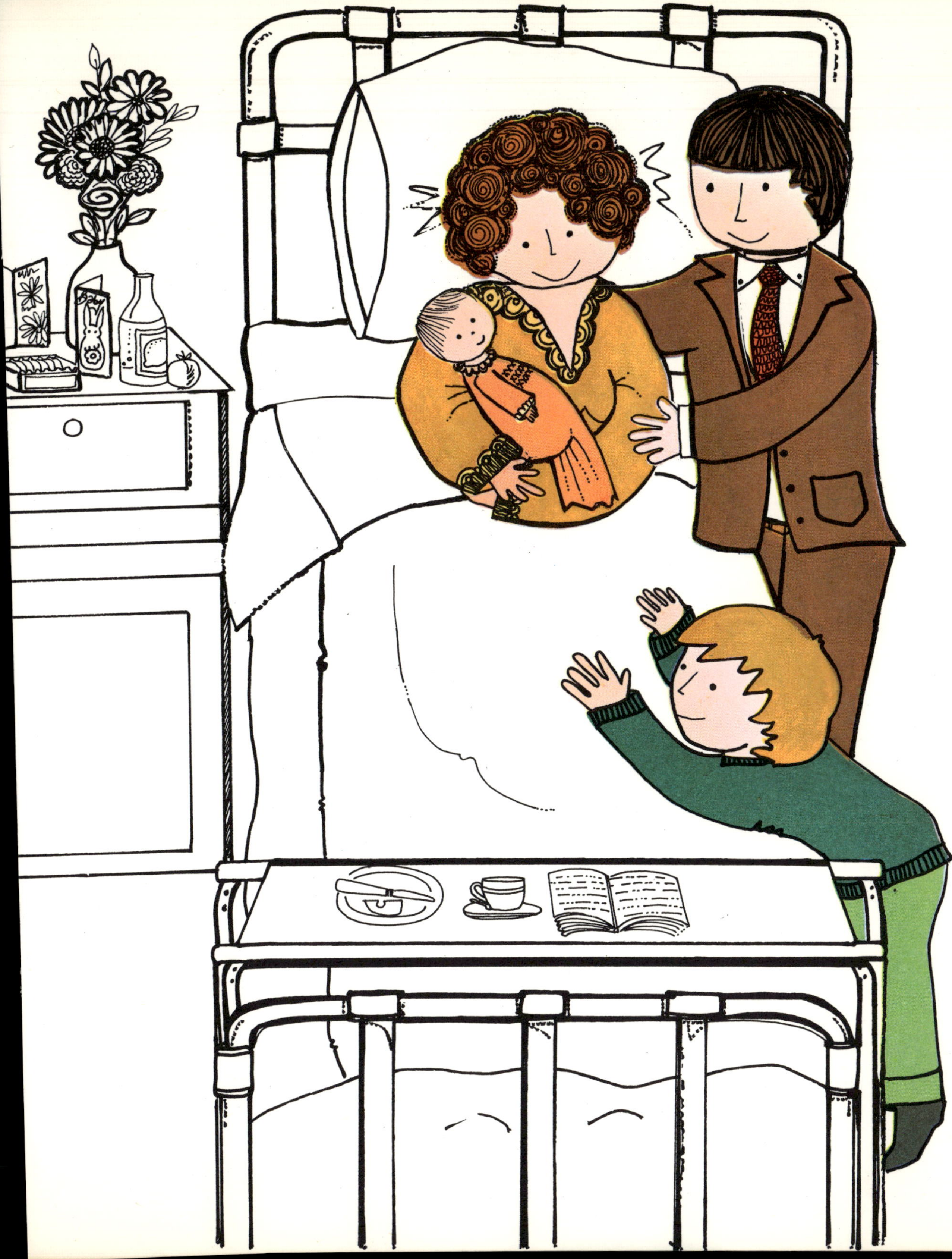